Aromatherapy

A Handbook of Aromatherapy and Essential Oils

Kelly Kohn

PUBLISHED BY:
Kelly Kohn

Disclaimer

The information contained in this book is for general information purposes only. The information is provided by the authors and while we endeavor to keep the information up to date and correct, we make no representations or warranties of any kind, express or implied, about the completeness, accuracy, reliability, suitability or availability with respect to the book or the information, products, services, or related graphics contained in the book for any purpose. Any reliance you place on such information is therefore strictly at your own risk.

Table of Contents

What is aromatherapy?

Aromatherapy is the art of using plant essences to bring about healing. The name is something of a misnomer as the medicine is from the active ingredients which work from inside the body. Whilst it is true that each of the oils has their own distinct aroma, most of the magic comes about in a very different way.

They can be used a number of ways. When inhaled essential oils release molecules which travel to the brain and work on a part of the brain called the limbic system. This is the area of the mind which affects emotions and memory. When the oils reach this part of the brain it alters moods, relaxing us, sedating us or uplifting us.

The oils also have the ability to absorb through the skin and into the blood stream. Their active ingredients can work in a variety of ways to bring about healing. This could be to ease pain, stimulate blood flow or even trigger hormonal changes. The list is endless.

When visiting a professional aromatherapist, you will go through a full question and answer session where they determine not just information about your presenting symptoms but also your job and also your lifestyle.

Many people use aromatherapy because they want some relief from stress in their lives. Certain essential oils will do a miraculous job in helping that, but the therapist will also help you to find ways to alleviate the stress you are feeling, to detoxify the effects it has had on your body and to show you how to nourish it back into health.

Most people will recognize aromatherapy as being used in massage. The effect of kneading and warming the muscles works very well in this medium. The oils though can be applied using a variety of means. A few drops of lavender oil for instance in the bath will encourage a good night's sleep. Sandalwood used the same way is aphrodisiac and conducive to romance.

Creams and lotions are also an excellent way of being able to have small doses of the oils little and often. These are best applied either to the affected part if the skin is not broken or alternatively on the inside of the wrist where there is an excellent blood supply. As the skin is very thin here, they absorb quickly helped by the close proximity of the warmth of the blood. Once in the system they will flush to the internal parts which need it. This is an effective way of applying a treatment for diarrhoea for instance.

Inhalations are good for decongesting blocked noses and these can be just a few drops in hot water to make unclogged your nose! These oils will also affect the mood in the room so you can buy essential oil burners which are little pots with candles below which keep the water warm contained within. Once the oils start to heat through, the molecules become wider apart and they are distributed into the atmosphere as gasses. This is a very potent way to manipulate your environment. It is perfect for relaxation, for seduction or even for helping your house to sell.

Where does the practice of aromatherapy come from?

Aromatherapy and the practice of using plant essences for health can be traced back many thousands of years. In excavations of the tombs in the Valley of the Kings, there have been discoveries of tears of frankincense and myrrh which was used in the embalming process. We can see references to plant knowledge in the Materia Medica, the only work by Pliny which was not destroyed by Vesuvius in AD 79. However it was not really until an Arab by the name of Abu Ali Ibn Cinna (or Avicenna to some) wrote works in AD 980 that we see true essential oils being used. Whilst it is unclear whether he invented the process of distillation, his works are the first we have seen with diagrams of the required equipment illustrated.

By medieval times every great house had a still room and the floral and herbal essences were being used extensively not only in herbal medicine but in cooking too. Some of the old theories still are with us in our lives today. The practice of eating mint with lamb for instance is to break down the fat and help digestion. When the crusaders came back to Britain from the Middle East they bought with them wonderful spices and resins which the Europeans had never before seen. Suddenly the range of products they could draw from was incredible.

As the 17th and 18th centuries rolled in, the Age of Reason took over and really the world pushed the old folklores back into the background as scientists began to understand more about our bodies. Science established how to extract the active ingredients from plants such as foxglove, valerian and poppies and make wonderful medicines such as digitalis, valium and morphine. The main effects of these plants were amazing supporting the heart and reducing unbearable pain. However that which brought about the wonderful healing to so many people brought tragic side effects of addiction and dependency too. .

Throughout the years there have always been fringe followings of the plants, those who stood true to the cause so to speak. In the early 20th Century a scientist by the name of Dr Jean Valnet was working in his lab and suffered a terrible burn on his hand. Plunging it into the first cold thing he could find, he stuck it into a vat of lavender oil. Very quickly the pain went away and over the coming days he was astounded at the rate in which the tissues healed. From that day on he devoted his life into promoting essential oils as a means of healing.

The sixties came and the hippy movement experimented with plants and their hallucinogenic effects but also made great steps forward in understanding how the physical body is inextricably linked to the mental and spiritual wellness. An understanding about the wholeness of a plant was gained and now we understand that the action of isolating one active ingredient from a plant is what can cause such potential health risks. The magic of the medicine is balanced within the plant in its entirety. By using the essences of the whole plant we alleviate the risk of dangerous side effects and instead enjoy the many main effects it has to offer.

Today aromatherapy has become a most complex medicine. Using essential oils we can bring about both physical healing and also emotional wellness too.

No longer a fringe science, a thousand years of research later, aromatherapy is very much a mainstream complementary medicine.

Is aromatherapy effective?

Aromatherapy uses the concentrated extracts of plants to bring about wellness in a person. They are very potent tools of healing. These are called essential oils and they have the ability to absorb through the skin and into the blood stream and then travel around the body system. In addition they are one of the only things known to many which have the ability to cross the blood brain barrier.

The oil is made up of many thousands of chemical constituents, molecules which determine the way any essential oil will react. Monoterpenes for instance are antibacterial but will also work as decongestants. Phenols are stimulating within the blood stream and sequiterpenes are antiallergenic.

Many people choose to use aromatherapy simply to affect their moods, choosing oils like lavender and camomile to soothe them or geranium to lift their spirit. There is a great more diversity of healing available.

The oils can be applied to the skin in a number of ways using a carrier to dilute their potency. Massage is a popular way, as is adding the oils to bathwater. Once in the blood stream the chemical constituents can get to work increasing immunity and balancing out any hormone irregularities there is.

Over the last twenty years it has been more and more accepted as a mainstream medicine. All of the time, more and more clinical trials are being conducted to find out to what degree oils will help varying conditions. Calendula oil for instance is now accepted to be the very best aid to healing for cancer radiation treatment burns. Melissa oil too is recognized as an extremely good aid for memory and behavior problems in patients with dementia.

Whilst it should not be used in replacement of any advice or medicine the doctor gives to you, it is an extremely useful complementary therapy. Having access to essential oil is like having a veritable hospital of medicines in one tiny bottle.   Aromatherapy is not simply effective it is like a sledge hammer to infection and warm blanket of a hug to low spirits.

How are essential oils extracted?

There are several processes of extracting essential oils from their plant matter dependant on how easily the host surrenders the chemical components.

By far the most common method of extracting essential oils is by distillation. It is not clear when this was first discovered but the works of an Arabian perfumer called Avicenna has pictures of stills in his writings from as early as AD 790.

To understand this process you must go back to your early science classes, to when you learned about the ways molecules are arranged in different states. They are most densely packed when they are solid, in fluid they are further apart and when in gas form they have large spaces between them and are able to move about most freely.

Fractional Distillation

The process of distillation relies on changing the molecule make up without changing the composition. That is to say, the chemical constituency remains intact even though it is changed to steam and fluid. Plant matter is collected into a still and steam is purged through it. As the water vapor passes through, it warms the matter and the oils are released into the steam. The vapor is then collected in another receptacle and is then cooled. The vapor returns to a water state. Since oil and water do not mix, the oil is left floating on top of the water. This is then separated off leaving two different products of the essential oil and the floral water (also known as a hydrosol) containing trace elements of the plant.

In some cases the oil is now left with some of the components missing. An example of this is Rose Otto oil which misses the alcohol which actually gives the oil its scent. This requires the oil to be distilled again to remove the alcohol which can then be added to the essential oil. This action is called cohobation.

Expression

Citrus oils in the main are extracted by a simple pressure on their peels. We call this expression. Most production is done via a method called écuelle à piquer which, roughly translated means poke with a spike. A rotating device uses a sharp needle to puncture the cells in the rind. The oil is then released into a receptacle. It is then necessary to separate off any extra water etc that has been collected by the process. This is a very cheap process for producers to undertake.

Solvent Extraction

Some people will argue that oils extracted by this method should not be used for aromatherapy as the plant essence created is not entirely pure. This method leaves a residue of between 6-20% behind and so the oil is quite severely contaminated. CO_2 extraction however does provide an extremely good quality and pure oil and the CO_2 of course dissipates almost completely at the end of the process.

Solvent extraction is mainly used when the plant matter does not easily give up its oil. Resins for example like frankincense and myrrh are extracted in this way. Other solvents to look out for are benzene and hexane which will create more inferior oils.

Enfleurage

This is a very ancient technique and although you can still find oils extracted by this method it is very costly to do and it is no longer part of mainstream production. It is used to draw oils out of petals which may be too delicate to withstand the rigors of distillation. Rose, Jasmine and Tuberose oils are usually the most used. To extract the essential oils great trays are smeared with vegetable fat and then lain out in the sun. They are covered with hundreds of petals and as the heat softens them the oils are released into the fat. The process is repeated time and again until the fat is entirely saturated with the plant's essence.

Then, to separate the oil from the fat, the concoction is washed with an alcohol which leaves behind the very finest, gorgeous essential oil.

How do you use aromatherapy essential oils?

Essential oils can be evaporated in a burner or can be used atopically, that is on the skin. Once they are on the skin they will absorb through it and flush through the blood stream. They must be diluted in some way. One lovely way to allow the oils to do their work is to put a few drops in your bath water. Muscles react to the warmth of water and begin to relax. The skin is the largest organ in the body and when you lie in the bath it means there are thousands of pores which allow the oils to enter the body.

The kneading of the fibers of the muscles warms them allows the essential oils to do their work. For this you must use some sort of carrier, generally that would be some kind of vegetable oil but it could also be talcum powder.

It is usually advisable to use a dilution of one drop of essential oils to 25 of carrier oil, but this is not an exact science.

It is worth noting that the body will take what it needs from the essential oils and the rest is excreted as waste. Since essential oils are expensive commodities it is worth remembering that less is more.

Useful carrier oils for massage are:

- Almond
- Sunflower
- Borage
- Jasmine
- Coconut Oils

What is meant by neat?

Whilst the large majority of essential oils should be diluted before they are applied to the skin there are some which can be used neat. This means that they can be used directly from the bottle and do not need to be mixed into something else. There are many different schools about when this is appropriate. Some disciplines of professional aromatherapy use a process called the Raindrop Technique where just one drop of the oil is used neat on the energy centre of the body.

Many oils however are what are called dermal irritants in concentration; that is they will irritate the skin. Some of them can give quite severe burns and also skin discoloration. For this reason using essential oils neat is very rarely advocated.

Here are the exceptions:
Both lavender and tea tree can be used neat on the skin.

Lavender poured neat onto a burn will very quickly take the sting out and stop damage going to the lower layers of skin.

Use either lavender or tea tree neat on a spot to kill the underlying infection and get rid of the breakout.

Lavender neat on the temples will quickly ease a headache. Rub undiluted tea tree onto the inside of the skin to prevent spread of a cold or flu infection.

One other trick is to use lemon neat on a wart or verrucae. This is a very powerful dermal irritant so this must be done with a cotton bud onto the affected part being careful not to touch any healthy skin. This is strong anti viral and will kill the virus within days.

Apart from these few ideas it is best to always use essential oils in a carrier of some kind. Whether that is a cream or lotion, in the bath or perhaps in massage oil, the oils are so concentrated there is little reason for them to be used neat.

What are the different ways by which you may apply aromatherapy?

There is a whole wealth of ways to use aromatherapy oils to bring about healing. Although some of the oils, lavender and tea tree can be used neat (that is undiluted) on the skin the rest require some kind of carrier.

Here are some of the best ways of using essential oils:

1. Bath
2. Massage
3. Evaporated Or Diffused Into The Atmosphere
4. Creams And Lotions
5. Compresses

In the bath

By far the most common way of using aromatherapy, this is a great way to enjoy a bit of pampering whilst the oils do their work.

In order to wave their magic wands the oils need to be able to get into the body. When you lie in the bath they can do this in two ways. The first is when the oils warm it causes them to change their state into gas. They evaporate into the steam of the bath and then you can very easily inhale them. They travel up to the brain via the sinuses which are the only nerves which go directly to the brain.

Once there they activate a part of the brain called the limbic system. This is the part which we use to make memories but it also affects our moods. The second way is via the skin which is the largest organ of our body.

When you lie in the bath it gives the oils an enormous surface area to go through. The warmth of the water opens the pores so that the oils can get through very quickly at a number of points. Once they enter into the blood stream and circulate around the body. The heart pumps the oils around and the body creates tiny chemical reactions as it goes.

Inside of the body the muscles also respond to the bath. The fibers relax from the warmth and they open allowing the oils far better access to heal.

The effects of using aromatherapy in the bath are really quite radical and take a very small requirement of oils. Around 5 drops is enough for one bath. The process of the oils entering into the system will take around 20 minutes so schedule enough time really to indulge!

Massage
Many people will associate the art of aromatherapy with massage and the two do go hand in hand. Whilst the essential oils do an excellent job of healing on their own, massage offers a whole new dimension to the healing.

The majority of the strokes in a massage are long and slow. A full body massage will take as much as an hour and a half to perform. The patient must lie still for a long time and relinquish complete control to the masseur. This is incredibly relaxing. Apart from smoothing strokes there is a requirement for more rigorous ones too. These encourage blood flow to the muscles and increase oxygen nutrients too.

To use essential oils for massage, you will need to use a carrier. Use any oil you have in the kitchen cupboard really but for relaxation you could try calendula or borage oils too. Many therapists will also add wheat germ oil to their mix as it increases the vibrancy contained in the oils and also fills the blend with Vitamin E.

Burning

This can be done by using aromatherapy candles or perhaps evaporators too. An evaporator has a bowl atop a candle usually. The bowl is filled with warm water and a few drops of oil are added. As the oils warm they evaporate into the air and bring about changes to the room. Use them for relaxation or also to help unblock noses.

Inhalations are most useful to either cleanse the skin or unblock congested sinuses.
Fill a bowl with just below boiling water and add your essential oils. Put your face around 6-8 inches away from the bowl and cover your head with a towel. The towel traps the steam around you a little like a sauna and then the oils get to work.

Be careful not to scald your skin though as the steam can become very hot.
The warmth of the steam encourages pores to open and body tissue to relax. This also means that catarrh will become thinner and begin to run.

In the case of skin care opening the pores allows the oils to get into the skin but also dirt to come out too. This is a very quick way to deep clean your skin.

Creams and lotions

This is a very useful way to use essential oils on a daily basis. It is only necessary for the oils to get into the system to be able to do their work. Work on the basis of around a 3 % dilution to a 97% base carrier. Skin care for instance works very well in this way. Consider mixing essential oils into moisturizers or masques, or perhaps for skin conditions such as eczema and psoriasis and ointment base may be used.

This can of course be extended to a whole range of possibilities, talc's, shampoos and gels all come immediately to mind.

How to make aromatherapy inhalations?

An aromatherapy inhalation is an excellent way to either treat sinus congestion or to cleanse the skin.

The oils vaporize very quickly and so have very quick access through the skin. It works in a very similar way to a mini steam room or sauna. To make an inhalation is so easy it is daft! Be aware though the steam is extremely hot and can scald if you are too close to the bowl. It is also not advisable for patients who exhibit high blood pressure as the warmth can bring about adverse reactions.

Pour just under boiling water into a large bowl and add essential oils. Take a large towel and place it over your head so it also comes down and covers the sides of the bowl. Keep your head around 6-8 inches away from the bowl to prevent scalding.

By trapping the steam around your face it forces the pores of the skin to open. Oils can get into the blood stream quickly to do their work. The gaseous molecules of the oils are also able travel up the nose to the sinuses and get to work breaking down the catarrh.

How to make aromatherapy room diffusions?

You may also see aromatherapy room diffusers called evaporators. The effect is the same. The process is to find a way which will allow essential oils to diffuse into the air and bring about changes. Usually this is done to change the mood of the room. You may want to have a serene atmosphere in the living room or one for seduction in the bedroom. Other times relaxation or focus may be the key.

There are many ways to bring this about. Here are some ideas.

Use a bowl of warm water

Often these are built into evaporators which you can buy but you can get the same effect by simply putting a bowl of water atop your radiator. The water stays warm and the oils will evaporate. One or two drops of oil are sufficient here.

Use a tissue

This method is limited as eventually all of the volatile molecules will evaporate and so the tissue will lose is potency. I find it useful however to throw a couple of tissues into waste paper bins to add a residual freshness to the room. Simply put one of two drops on the tissue and allow them to evaporate.

Light bulb diffusers

These ceramic rings are designed to sit on top of light bulbs. They are extremely porous so any oil which you add is simply drawn into the clay. The heat of the lamp in the evening activates the oils encouraging them evaporate and diffuse into the air. It is usually sufficient to use just one of two drops or perhaps dilute in a ¼ teaspoon of water.

Tealights

It is possible to buy tealights which contain essential oils. However if you decide to use a normal candle, simply wait until the wax is melted a little and drop one drop of essential oil into the liquid wax.

Here are some ideas of oils which work well in diffusers:

For relaxation
Lavender, camomile, frankincense, vertivert, patchouli and geranium

For romance
Sandalwood, jasmine, ylang ylang

For merriment
Use bergamot, mandarin or lemon grass (lemongrass and citronella are great for repelling inspects too....think BBQ!)

For focus in study
Rosemary and rosewood

For prayer
Frankincense or Angelica

To unblock sinuses
For sinus congestion choose oils such as eucalyptus camphor, myrrh, galbanum and frankincense. To cleanse the skin use oils such as carrot seed, cypress, myrtle or Oakmoss Eucalyptus

It is also possible to buy electrical diffusers too. These have the added benefit of having no concern about exposed flames.

How do you make mood enhancers aromatherapy candle?

Aromatherapy candles can make wonderful mood enhancers. They can facilitate changes which we would not have dreamed possible. From the everyday relaxation at the end of the day to helping your home to sell, how to make aromatherapy candles is a skill which everyone should learn how to do.

The easiest way is with a sheet of beeswax which you can buy from most craft shops or direct from a beekeeper.

The sheets come in rectangular shapes and you can get 4 candles from each one. Cut the rectangle in half vertically and then cut each section diagonally to create two triangles.

Choose which essential oil you want to use according to the effects you want it to have.
Lavender, camomile and geranium are relaxing for example. For a more convivial atmosphere you could try mandarin, orange, lemon or bergamot. Seductive candles are best created with sandalwood or ylang ylang. Experiment to find which ones you likes the most.

Smear some essential oil down the vertical edge of your triangle. Let it dry for a few moments then take a piece of cotton string and make yourself a wick. Lay it along the same vertical side and now crease a small line of the beeswax against the wick.

Now, tightly roll the beeswax around the wick, winding it as tightly as you can against the string. Trim the wick to length.

Some people prefer to put the essential oil directly onto the wick but as it burns you lose the freshness of the scent that way.

How to make aromatherapy baths?

An aromatherapy bath must surely be the perfect end to the day. It is simple to make time for, costs very little money and is the perfect way to pamper yourself or show someone you care.

All that is required is to fill the bath with warm water then add 5-10 drops of the desired oil. Essential oils all bring about different effects so here are some ideas of ones which you could choose.

For relaxation use lavender, although one of the cheaper oils on the market it is tremendously efficient in reducing stress and relaxing muscles. This oil will also make you very sleepy so it is a great oil to use at bedtime.

Camomile too, is very restful. It will also reduce cramps and pain, so it is very helpful for period pains or tummy ache.

For back ache I would still use lavender but also add juniper too.

For days when the life seems incredibly hard a bottle of geranium oil is the best friend you can get.

A very effective way to make an aromatherapy bath is to run it hot and add the oils and then go out and leave the door closed for a while. This amasses steam and fills the air of the bathroom with the essential oil molecules. Ensure the bathwater is adequately cooled before you climb in.

When inhaled, essential oils have a very fast journey to the brain. There, they circulate and trigger actions in a part of the brain called the limbic system which is responsible for the formation and storage of memories. As it regulates our emotions too, very quickly our mind begins to relax.

At the same time the warm water does two different things to our body. It opens the pores of the skin allowing the oils to draw through and it relaxes the muscles too. Once inside of the body the oils flush around the blood stream affecting the body systems as they go.

In total it takes around 20 minutes for the skin to go through the full process of osmosis and for the blood to become full of the oils. Languish for at least that long!

How to make aromatherapy compresses?

Aromatherapy compresses area very effective way of allowing on particular part of the skin to open to allow access for essential oils to get in. Examples may be warm compresses to help earache or perhaps back pain in Pre-Menstrual Tension (PMT). Cold compresses are helpful to reduce the bleeding from a wound. A mixture of warm and cold compresses will allow the pores of the skin to open and close making a suction effect. This is extremely helpful for drawing out toxins in the body, for example for treatment of an abscess.

To make a compress fill a bowl with water, hot water for a warm compress (not as hot as it could scald the skin) and cold water otherwise.

Add the essential oils to the water and mix well to break up the oils.

Soak a flannel in the water for a minute or so. This could be a small bud of cotton wool or even a full size beach towel depending on the size of the area you want to treat.

Wring it out well and place on the area affected.

In total it takes about 20 minutes for the process of osmosis to complete and draw the essential oils through the skin. Leave for the full amount of time.

If hot and cold compresses are to be used together, ensure that the patient is covered with a towel as they can become very cold.

After use ensure that all cloths used for the compresses are thoroughly washed out. The salts which are drawn from the tissues of the body can very quickly rot the fabric.

How to make use of aromatherapy in massages?

Using aromatherapy to enhance the effects of massage is an extremely efficient aid to healing. The action of the kneading of the muscles makes it very simple for the oils to gain entry and start doing their magic. Adding essential oils to massage will help to increase relaxation, stimulate blood flow, remove toxins and relax even further still.

For extra relaxation use oils such as lavender, camomile, geranium or patchouli; these are not only physically relaxing but emotionally soothing too. For patients who find it difficult to relax in their treatment, add frankincense to the blend. This will slow their breathing allowing them to submit to the calm.

For muscle pain use the same oils as above but also add ones to manage toxicity in the fibrous tissue. Juniper is wonderful for breaking down toxins and flushing them away. Black pepper encourages circulation and encourages good blood flow. Cypress will invigorate the muscles too.

For menstrual tension essential oils are particularly useful. While massaging over the abdomen during the first two days of the period is painful, a simple stroking in of the oils allows them to address bloating and pain. Consider using rose, jasmine or geranium here.

While massage may be contraindicated in conditions like sciatica, rosemary can replace soothing strokes. It is a specific for nerve pain and is an excellent substitution in therapy.

Massage also helps to remove toxicity by stimulating lymphatic drainage. Oils which will enhance this action are fennel, grapefruit and again cypress. These are helpful in PMT bloating but also in the treatment of cellulite too.

Perhaps massage may also be used to improve intimacy in a relationship, a romantic wind down before bed. Lovely seductive oils can really enhance this. Choose ylang ylang, sandalwood, patchouli or jasmine oils.

Essential oils are extremely potent. Use a consistency of 3% essential oils to 97% carrier in a blend.

Which essential oils are good to blend?

Blending essential oils is an art which perfumers have worked for centuries to perfect. In aromatherapy the endeavor is to find a blend which both smells wonderful but also brings about the best healing results. This is called a synergistic blend.

In a well performing synergistic blend, the different parts of the mix work together to enhance each of the others' healing abilities.

This is done through a process known as blending notes. The note of the oil is dependent on its volatility; that is how quickly it evaporates. The top or head notes evaporate quickest and tend to be sharp citrusy scents. These are uplifting and refreshing.

The oils which are less volatile are called the middle or heart notes and their job is to balance the blend. The slowest and thus the deepest smelling notes are called the base notes. These linger long after the top parts of the blend have evaporated.

Here are some ideas of which oils fit where into the list

Base notes

Angelica, Peru Balsam, Benzoin, Cedarwood Atlas, Cedarwood Virginian, Frankincense, Helichrysum, Myrrh, Oakmoss, Patchouli, Sandalwood, Spikenard, Vanilla, Vetiver

Middle

Anise, Basil, Bay Laurel, Bergamot, Bergamot Mint, Boronia, Citronella, Eucalyptus, Galbanum, Grapefruit, Lemon, Lemongrass, Lime, Mandarin, Myrtle, Lemon, Orange, Bitter Orange, Sweet Peppermint, Petitgrain, Ravensara, Spearmint, Tagetes, Tangerine, Tuberose, ylang ylang

Top

Bay, Rosewood, Cajuput, Cardamom, Carrot Seed, Chamomile, German, Chamomile, Roman, Cinnamon, Clary Sage, Clove, Coriander, Cypress, Dill, Elemi, Eucalyptus, Lemon, Eucalyptus Radiata, Fir Needle, Geranium, Geranium, Rose, Hyssop, Jasmine, Juniper Berry, Kanuka, Linden Blossom, Manuka, Marjoram, May Chang/Litsea Cubeba, Neroli, Niaouli, Nutmeg, Oregano, Palmarosa, Parsley, Pepper, Black, Pine, Rose, Rosemary, Rosewood, Spruce, Tea Tree, Thyme, Violet Leaf, Yarrow.

To mix blends try to take equal numbers of each of the oils from each list to make a good balance of notes. When you achieve this balance you will be able to smell it in the blend. Consider the experience as if it were sound. When a harmony is correct it is pleasing to the ear. A chord made up of notes which are separated by just one in between work best, for example A,C,E. Likewise in colors, put two shades which are similar together and they tend to look clashing, red and fuchsia for instance.

It is usual to find that in blending, less is more. Use no more than 2 of each set to create a really effective blend.

How do you store your essential oils properly?

Essential oils should be kept on dark bottles out of the reach of little fingers. Over time they can begin to degrade through a process called oxidation. This can be delayed by keeping the oils in a cool dark place.

Where should you store your essential oils?

Keep your dark glass bottles either in a drawer or a sealable box to contain the vapors from the bottles. This makes it far easier to quickly find the oils you require in therapy.

How can you be sure you are purchasing good, quality essential oils?

Since essential oils can very much vary in price it can be difficult to be reassured that you are buying good quality and effective oils. One of the main things to look for is the labeling on the bottles to give you some clues.

A reputable essential oil dealer will always label their oils with both the English name and the Latin name too. This is what is known as binomial nomenclature. The first word gives you the family of plants the oil came from and the second word (which should not have a capital letter) tells you the species it is specific to.

In the United States you will often see essential oils listed as Grade A, this is part of a set of four grades meaning grade A is what is termed therapeutic grade, that is to say the purest. In actual fact this is grading system which is purely touted by MLM marketing companies and no such official legislation exists.

In France there is also a governing body called AFNOR who issue grading to oils produced there. This is for a slightly different reason as they are largely concerned with the economic impact that export of essential oils can bring to their country.

The ways which oils have been extracted can also be a factor. Those which have been obtained through solvent extraction will be less pure than those obtained by distillation as solvents will leave a residue. It is worth looking out for oils which have been obtained by CO_2 extraction, although costly these will have less residual contamination.

Sometimes contamination can be deliberate too. If you see a bottle of rose oil which seems very cheap for example, it is worth checking the label to see if it has been mixed with oil. Often you may see a 5% dilution in a carrier oil perhaps.

Similarly some essential oils are "cut" with another cheaper oil to make the price less expensive. A good example of this Lemon Balm oil of Melissa officinalis. Look for Melissa (True) on labels which means there is an absence of lemongrass in the mix.

Essential oils do have a shelf life to them. A process called oxidation means that after a period of time they lose their effects and begin to go rancid. Citrus oils for example have very short shelf lives. Look for clues as to how long the retailer has had the oils on the shelf. For this reason you may find larger retailers a better source to buy from.

Oils should also always be kept in a dark bottle and also out of direct sunlight. Again this is because of the oxidation process. Head for suppliers which have got their stores at the back of the shop.

Lastly price is a big indicator. Aromatherapy is a very fiercely competitive market and anyone who really overprices their oils will be left behind. Conditions affect harvests as of course do other factors outside of the producer's control, diesel for shipping or export duties to name just a few. This means that prices of essential oils do fluctuate, but in the scheme of things really, not that much. If the oil looks to be much cheaper than you have seen recently on the market, the chances are it is not as likely to be of very good quality.

Using Essential Oils Safely

Why is aromatherapy not appropriate for everyone?

While a wonderfully effective method of healing, aromatherapy is not for everyone. The chemical constituents of the oils can bring about myriad effect, some quite detrimental to health and in some conditions use of the oils is not advisable.

Cancer patients should avoid aromatherapy. The oils stimulate many of the bodies systems and there are some oils which may encourage tumors to grow.

Patients with hemophilia are advised not to use the oils either, for fear of thinning the blood more.

People with diabetes should use caution as many of the oils work on the endocrine system. One of the sets of glands contained is called the Islets of Langerhans which is part of the pancreas. This manufactures insulin. Any oils triggering this area could compromise the body's ability to metabolize sugar effectively. In some cases this can be severe enough to even induce coma. Aromatherapy should not be used in the first 16 weeks of pregnancy.

Many of the oils contain constituents which can act as neurotoxins so patients suffering from epilepsy should use with care as should those exhibiting delusional traits for example schizophrenia.

What are some of the side-effects of aromatherapy?

There are no side effects to aromatherapy; however the oils themselves have many main effects. When choosing oil for a blend it is important to look at ALL the actions it is capable of. Take rosemary oil for example. It is by far the most effective oil that you can find for helping nerve pain. It is wonderful for enhancing memory too. It has the ability to lower cholesterol and is wonderful for digestive complaints. It is invigorating especially to the circulatory system and for this reason is being researched for its efficacy for helping to reduce hair loss. Given all of these reasons rosemary is quite a wonder oil to use. Everyone will love it but it also has active constituents called ketones which in patients with epilepsy can cause seizures.

Aromatherapy is built on the principle that using the whole plant is what brings about wellness. Science over the decades has learned just how effective plants can be for healing and have synthesized components to make life saving drugs. Digitalis, valium and morphine all originated from plant extracts. As a therapy, isolating these properties and breaking down the plants are what cause side effects such as dependency and addiction.

Why should essential oils be not applied on broken skin?

Oils applied to broken skin can cause serious skin sensitivity. Always apply them in carrier oil and never over the broken area. The oils are able to absorb through the skin and into the blood stream which means as long as they are applied to the body they will find their own way to the part of the body which needs them.

Why should aromatherapy oil be not applied directly to the skin?

Essential oils used in aromatherapy are extremely potent and should not be applied directly to the skin. The essences are so concentrated that some of them even have the ability to burn the skin and can irritate it so badly.

Others are what are called phyto toxic meaning they will react with light. Citrus oils in particular will trigger the body to manufacture melanin and will make the skin go brown where the oil has been added.

It is important to recognize just how powerful these oils are and to accept there really is no need to apply them in such large amounts. By diluting them not only do you preserve your skin but you also allow your oil supply to last longer, saving you money as you go!

Should you seek immediate medical attention if the essential oil is accidentally ingested?

If someone accidentally ingests essential oils, it is very important to seek medical advice. Take the empty bottle with you to the hospital so that the doctor can assess any potential problems.

Many of the oils will have been extracted from food sources in the first place, coriander, lemon or peppermint for example. In such high concentration the oils can have really quite detrimental effects. Some can cause hallucinations, other heavy bleeding or even can irritate the digestive tract.

Try to assess how much they have taken. As essential oils are so concentrated it actually taste, in some cases rather unpleasant so it is rare that some drink very much…but of course it can happen.

It is worth getting them to drink a large amount of milk before they get to the hospital to dilute the mix but also to line the stomach ready for any potential stomach pumping which may be required.

Given the severity of any risks imposed it should require no instruction that care be taken that essential oils be stored out of reach of little fingers.

Is there any essential oil safe to use for people with epilepsy?

Some essential oils contain neurotoxins which can be convulsant to people with epilepsy. Oils to avoid are Rosemary, Fennel, Sage and Hyssop. Nutmeg also has psychotropic effects. Other oils which have compounds containing thujone which can be convulsant too, these are Thuja, Lavendula latifolia or spike lavender, Tansy and Wormwood.

Historically aromatherapists would avoid treating patients with epilepsy for fear they may experience a seizure. In fact this very rarely happens. Recent research by the Queen Elizabeth Hospital in Birmingham (UK) shows that using essential oils and massage to reduce the effects of stress can actually help to minimize the frequency of fitting.

It is important to avoid the oils listed above but apart from these there are no other concerns to be considered. Oils can be chosen freely.

Patients with epilepsy do have a slightly altered sense of smell and so they tend to veer towards sweeter smelling oils. It has been shown that used in massage jasmine and ylang ylang offer real benefits to epilepsy sufferers.

Why should pregnant and lactating mothers avoid using essential oil?

Essential oils are a wonderful help in regulating hormones but pregnant and lactating mothers should use oils with care. Essential oils travel through the skin and into the blood stream and during pregnancy have the ability to affect baby too.

During the delicate first trimester it is advised that no essential oils be used. For nausea and morning sickness many women find herbal teas to be of just effective use. From 16 weeks onwards some more delicate oils may be introduced.

- Citrus oils, such as tangerine and Neroli
- Chamomile matricaria
- Lavender
- Frankincense
- Black pepper
- Peppermint
- Ylang ylang
- Eucalyptus
- Bergamot
- Cypress
- Tea tree oil
- Geranium
- Spearmint

While aromatherapy prides itself in having no side effects, essential oils instead have many main effects. While some are relaxing or invigorating they can just as likely promote heavy bleeding, hemorrhage or miscarriage. They are very potent things, many being uterine tonics or stimulating hormones from the endocrine system.

In the later terms of pregnancy, aromatherapists use these facts to their advantage. During labor clary sage and jasmine can increase contractions for instance. Used earlier in pregnancy this could cause dire effect but in the long and slow hours of labor this can be a blessing indeed.

After the stress of labor is all over, essential oils such as rose and geranium are wonderful for bringing mums hormones back into line. Carrot seed oil can stimulate milk production and Tagetes compresses are bliss to engorged breasts. There is a concern to be addressed though. Timing of the use of these oils is important as used to closely to feeding time baby can taste them. Some (Tagetes for instance) are very bitter and may discourage good feeding habits.

Is there any essential oil safe for pregnant and lactating mothers to use?

While there are many oils which are listed as safe during pregnancy they should all be used with care and never within the first trimester of pregnancy.

- Citrus oils, such as tangerine , mandarin and Neroli
- Chamomile matricaria
- Lavender
- Frankincense
- Black pepper
- Peppermint
- Ylang ylang
- Eucalyptus
- Bergamot
- Cypress
- Tea tree oil
- Geranium
- Spearmint

Oils which are useful in labour are Jasmine and Clary sage which help to strengthen contractions. It is not advisable to use these until labour has begun.

All the oils above are safe to lactating mothers. I would also add that Rose and Calendula officinalis are good too. Rose will help to balance the hormones after delivery. Calendula helps to heal the skin of cracked nipples. Be aware though, the taste of the essential oils will translate into the mother's milk and maybe unpleasant to the infant.

Actions of Essential Oils

Which essential oils have antibacterial properties?

In 2000 The Journal for Microbial Chemotherapy published a paper of their findings of essential oils and their antibacterial properties. A total of 14 oils were tested in petri dishes to assess their reactions in the fight against bacterial infections. The various strains of Staphylococcus , influenza and E Coli were all exposed to the rigours in turn of Cinnamon Bark, Lemongrass, Perilla, Thyme (wild) , Thyme (red), Thyme (geraniol) , Peppermint , Tea tree, Coriander, Lavender (spike), Lavender (true), Rosemary, Eucalyptus (radiata), and Lemon oils.

Across the board, all of them showed some degree of anti bacterial activity, but by far the most effective were cinnamon bark, Red and Wild Thyme and Lemongrass which inhabited every one of the six different strains tested. Tea tree also fared extremely well in the fight against E Coli. The two oils which showed the least activity in the strains were lemon and Eucalyptus radiata.

To the list of essential oils I would recommend for antibacterial properties Manuka, Niaouli, Ravensara and also Oregano.

Most of the oils on the list exhibit some degree of capability for dermal irritancy so I would always recommend dilution for these. The very best carrier to fight off in faction will be a very light lotion with the oils mixed in a dilution of around 1% essential oils and 99% carrier. A small amount applied regularly to the inside of the arm will start to fight off infection very quickly.

These oils would also work very well as a cleaning agent for surfaces to rid the home of germs too.

Which essential oils are adrenal stimulating?

One of the key problems in managing stress is that over time our adrenal glands become exhausted from all of the external pressures stimulating them for an extended amount of time. Essential oils can help here.

In the fight against stress, rather than finding oils which will stimulate the adrenals, we want ones which will boost them. I will explain why.

The adrenals are small glands which sit at atop our kidneys. Their job is to secrete a variety of different hormones. The one which we are primarily concerned with here is adrenaline. This hormone is what gives us our edge and keeps us safe in times of danger. It rules what is called our "fight and flight" syndrome.

This raises our heart rate and breathing and fills our muscles with oxygen to strengthen them in the fight we see before us. Now in the times of our ancestors this was very useful because it allowed us to outrun the saber tooth tiger, slay it and eat it.

When the feasting was over, he slept and the adrenaline levels could return to their resting levels. Today however we live under so many pressures the levels never quite return to normal. This over stimulation is what makes us feel burned out.

The oils which support the adrenal glands are Mandarin and Camomile maroc. These help to strengthen the adrenals and allow them to begin working effectively again.

The adrenals work in tandem with other glands in the endocrine system, (mainly the pituitary gland) and also the liver.

Oils which help to support the liver are rosemary, peppermint and eucalyptus. The pituitary should be supported using nutmeg oil.

I would advocate a blend of oils in a home treatment cream or lotion which can be applied very regularly, perhaps as often as three times a day on the inside of the arm. This gives the opportunity of the essential oils to stimulate the healing mechanisms which will very quickly have the adrenals functioning effectively.

Which essential oils act as vasodilators?

Vasodilator essential oils work in a very similar way to a very rigorous exercise work out. They encourage the blood vessels to open much wider so the blood becomes engorged with oxygen. This has two main effects. The skin then takes on a very healthy plumped up appearance but it also brings about this wonderful feeling of wellness a bit like the runners high.

There are three essential oils which act as true vasodilators and these are marjoram, geranium and also ylang ylang oils. Geranium can also be very effectively used for reducing the amount of redness in the cheeks which comes from rosacea for the same reason. Ylang ylang is able to reduce blood pressure too through its vasodilatory expression.

Complementary oils to add to blends are lemon, myrtle, cypress, black pepper and lemongrass. All of these will stimulate circulation and encourage good supply.
The best methods of application will be different according to the effects you want to bring. Most people would want good muscle strength. For this it would be best to utilize the benefits of a massage. The kneading and pummelling will add to the oxygenation of the muscles and further enhance their effects. The oil drop to the bath water too would be very effective. I would not use black pepper, lemongrass or lemon in this way as they are a little harsh on the skin. Cypress may be a little too invigorating before bed but geranium, ylang, ylang, myrtle and marjoram will also have the added benefits of bringing excellent sleep

For rosacea, add to your daily moisturiser. As many applications of ylang ylang as you can find will help lower blood pressure, blend it into massage oils, creams and lotions and also drip it into the bath.

Aromatherapy for the Body

Does aromatherapy calm and relax the body?

People potentially use aromatherapy for its ability to relax and calm more than for any other reason. The essential oils are able to do a very good job alone but when mixed with the soothing strokes of a massage, it can become absolutely sedative bliss.

The body is a complex machine taking directions entirely from the brain. Essential oils are able to absorb through the skin and into the blood stream and work in a way that allows the body to let go of tension and begin to relax.

First we need to look at what causes tension in the body which is usually the effects of stress. When we feel under pressure or experience anxiety or fear, our bodies secrete a hormone called adrenaline. This causes our heart rates to go faster and our breathing to speed up too. You may recognize how we clench the muscles in our shoulders and fists in particular but also our legs and buttocks too (mainly because of a natural response for the body to want to run away from the situation).

When a muscle has been over worked for a period of time it can no longer manage the bi product lactic acid which is left behind. Over time it becomes crystallized and gets knotted into the muscle fibers. Perhaps you have felt this giveaway crunching when you roll your neck?

Essential oils such as lavender and camomile are very soothing not only to the muscles but also to our frazzled nerves. Marjoram sends out messages right across the central nervous system for the organs to calm down.

Juniper is extremely good at breaking down the toxicity which is left in the joints and muscles leaving them clean and refreshed. The muscles fibers are then able to slip across each other easily making movement far less painful and easier.

Many people like to use aromatherapy oils in the bath to relax the body too. This is an excellent way to get them into the blood stream quickly. The water relaxes the muscles and opens the pores. It also gives a very large surface area into which the oils can absorb. This is both extremely relaxing to the body and calming to the mind.

Which aromatherapy oil is the best to use for massage to alleviate body pain?

Pain in the body can come from a variety of sources and aromatherapy oils can help reduce the agony you feel. By far the most effective pain killers you can find are lavender and camomile oils. Lavender you can use neat on the body and camomile must be diluted.

Often pain in the body will come from a buildup of toxicity which the body has not been able to rid itself of. This could come from over exertion in exercise or from the physical effects of stress for example. These toxins will eventually turn crystalline making it more difficult for the fibers to slip over each other easily. This friction causes pain. Juniper oil is wonderful for braking down this toxicity and flushing it out of the body.

Similarly the pain may result from nerve pain, headache, toothache or sciatica perhaps. Use of rosemary reduces the surges of agony this can produce and alleviates pain.

Care must however be taken with use of rosemary as it is high in neurotoxins which are able to induce fitting in people who are sufferers of epilepsy.

Tendons which have become stressed and torn over time can find help from frankincense oil. It restores elasticity to the fibers and helps them to regain strength.

All of these essential oils work well when dropped into the bath at the end of a long day. About 5 drops is plenty enough to fill the bath water. Massage too can be very helpful as the muscles are kneaded and warmed to stimulate them too.

Blend around 5 drops of oil into a 10 ml of carrier oil to create a blend. Carrier oils can be any vegetable oil that you find in your kitchen cupboard but very effective ones are calendula or borage.

Any good aromatherapy recipes for physical wellness?

(Amounts are numbers of drops to use)
Aphrodisiac massage oil – Jasmine x 2, ylang ylang x 2, Sandalwood x 2 in 25 ml of carrier oil

For nerve pain – Rosemary – Frankincense x 2 Rosemary x1 Lavender x 3 blended into 25ml of body lotion
To use for muscle training-   Cedarwood atlas x 2, black pepper x1, Juniper x 3 in 25 mml of body lotion

To alleviate bugs and germs – Tea tree x 2, Manuka x1, Kanuka x 2, Ravensara x 1, Niaouli x 1 and Elemi x1 mixed into 25 ml of body lotion and applied often as you remember on the inside of the arm.

Aromatherapy for the Mind

How does aromatherapy affect the person's mood?

Aromatherapy works on two very different systems within the body. Essential oils have the ability to absorb through the skin and into the blood stream. Once there they circulate around the blood stream and travel to the places which need them.

They can also be taken to the brain via the sinuses; that is they can be inhaled. For the most part oils will be inhaled because they are in evaporator or perhaps in a bath but the heat allows the oils to turn to gas and travel up the patient's nose. This is a very fast journey as the sinuses are the only nerves which go directly to the brain.

Scientific trials have recently proved that essential oils have the ability to cross the blood brain barrier and when their molecules reach the brain they affect an area called the limbic system. This is the part of our brain which not only governs our emotions but our memory too. With this is mind it can be that a memory from long ago can be triggered by a simple smell from the past.

The chemical constituents of an oil vary from plant to plant. Oils which contain components called sesqiterpenes have the ability to uplift the mood, while those containing esters (like camomile, and valerian for instance) are more likely to sedate.

Used in massage too the effects are further enhanced by the warming and relaxing of the muscles. The process of being touched is very nurturing and can promote a feeling of deep well being.

Which aromatherapy oil is the best for treating anxiety?

Long term anxiety can be detrimental to health. Using aromatherapy not only eases the mind but also reduces the physical after effects which can result on the body.

Geranium oil is the powerhouse when treating anxiety. Best used 5 drops in warm bathwater it quickly helps to lift the anxiety away.

Frankincense is a very ancient oil which has been used since time immemorial to induce a meditative state. It slows down the breath which in turn allows all of the other body processes to follow suit. It is relaxing to the muscles and very sedative too.

Lavender is soothing and a relatively cheap oil to buy. Apart from relaxing the mind and body it will also aid restful sleep.

The deep and musky tones of vertivert and patchouli make them wonderfully soothing oils. They will both calm the mind and also release tension from the muscles.

There are times though when anxiety can come from a short sharp shock and that can really induce panic. A drop of camphor really helps to alleviate trauma. It is a very strong oil and should be used with care, one drop in any treatment and no more.

Massage is by far the most effective method of using aromatherapy to treat anxiety. The actual process of doing nothing for an hour and a half is really quite difficult to do. It is the admission to yourself that the world won't just stop if you do. This is extremely conducive to healing.

Touch is a very soothing thing too and while the therapist kneads your muscles and calms away your stress the essential oils can set to healing your mind and body too.

How can aromatherapy fight off depression?

Aromatherapy uses the concentrated essences of plants to bring about changes in the mind and the body. Essential oils are one of the only things known be able to cross the blood brain barrier. Once there they are able work on a part of the mind called the limbic system. This controls not only our emotions but also our memory too.

Depression has many different symptoms and while aromatherapy can certainly help to alleviate these, medical guidance from your doctor should be sought. Here are some ideas of oils which will help.

Use uplifting oils to help to improve your mind. Oils such are **bergamot, geranium, melissa and cypress** are all wonderful for moving the gloom.

Research has shown that the amount of light we get on a daily basis affects not only our moods but our physical body too. A gland called the pineal is responsible for manufacturing hormones melatonin, which regulates sleep, and also serotonin, which affects mood, learning, intimacy and also many of our digestive process. If you find you feel withdrawn or unable to connect emotionally this could be a source of your problems. This particularly is true of people suffering from Seasonal Affective Disorder. Incidentally we know that women are more than 70% more likely to suffer from this condition and to suffer connected symptoms. Oils which can help boost your pineal are: **Lavender, Sandalwood, Frankincense, Parsley and Pine.**

Anxiety and hopelessness are best treated by the doctor especially if they present on a longer term basis. **Geranium and rose** are helpful as well as **mandarin and myrtle** oils. **Clary sage** is incredibly sedative and allows you to distance yourself emotionally from the problems. Use this oil with care; be aware that it does not mix well with alcohol as it can cause delusion.

Using Aromatherapy like a Pro...

How to treat insomnia with aromatherapy?

Treating insomnia with aromatherapy needs to be a two pronged approach.

While there are oils which will certainly soothe and relax you into a deep and restful sleep it is also necessary to tackle the reason why you are struggling to sleep in the first place.

One of the main protagonists is caffeine. Drinking tea and coffee can ramp your brain speeds up making it hard to settle at night.

Often stress can be a factor, or even being over tired. The best essential oil to help this is **marjoram oil**. It works on the central nervous system and stops the mind from keeping on going over things. Essential oils are able to affect not just emotional changes but also physical ones too. The marjoram will soothe the mind but also ease the muscles which are cramping in response to the stress.

By far the most effective oils for soothing are **Lavender and Camomile**. They are lovely in a slow soothing massage but equally as beneficial by having a few drops in the bath.

Often just the process of taking time out to pamper yourself will help you feel a little more relaxed but the oils themselves can do magical things. Used in the bath the oil molecules turn to vapor and are inhaled slowing down the breathing and reducing heart rate. The warmth of the water also relaxes the muscles and opens the pores for the oils to absorb through. Once in the blood stream they circulate around the body, relaxing and soothing as they go.

Another lovely way to help you drop off is to have an essential oils evaporate in your room. This is a gorgeous way to ensure your mind stays calm throughout the night. There is a consideration here though that you could fall asleep and the candle be left unattended. Ensure it is placed well away from curtains or anything which could cause a hazard.

Other oils which will help to relax are **Frankincense** which will slow down the breathing and bring about a very tranquil dreamlike state. For days when the world has really given you a kicking I recommend **Geranium** oil to let the day just lift away. **Spikenard, valerian** and **hop** oils help a great deal. You could also try replacing your teas and coffee with herbal teas made from these plants.

The most important aspect of tackling insomnia though is a good bedtime routine. Avoid going to bed too late and try to create a system of actions which you do each night. This way the body learns a new habit of going to sleep. The range of options is many. Whether you choose to languish in a luxurious aromatherapy bath or burn essential oils as you snuggle down with a good book, within days you will see an improvement in your insomnia.

How to treat allergies with aromatherapy?

Aromatherapy offers a number of lovely treatments which can help to soothe the symptoms of allergies. Usually if you were to visit a professional aromatherapist they would try to get to the root causes of the problem. The triggers which can make allergies rear their heads are too diverse to cover here and so I shall simply look at ones which can help alleviate the suffering they bring.

The most important oil in the fight against allergic reactions is **Lemon balm;** you may see this listed as **Melissa**. This oil is a natural antihistamine and will help to lower the problems you suffer.

Many outbreaks can present itching and soreness and for these I would suggest using **Lavender and Camomile**. This is both effective for skin breakouts but also the irritations in the sinus caused by irritants such as pollen.

In the case of hay fever the irritation to the sinuses will also cause congestion and for this I would suggest using **frankincense** which will unblock the nose.

In conditions such as eczema and psoriasis there can also be a very painful side issue of scratching breaking the skin. In particular this is a problem with children who suffer from eczema. For this I would suggest using **Myrrh** which is a very good skin healer and will help to protect and repair the cracks. For all of these conditions I would suggest using a cream or lotion to apply, for skin outbreaks apply to the affected area. For hay fever and sinus irritation rub a blend of oils over the cheekbones and forehead for a very fast absorption into the sinuses. This allows the aromatherapy treatment get a very fast and targeted attack on the symptoms of the allergies.

How to treat stress with aromatherapy?

Stress is probably the main way which people discover aromatherapy. The oils are so good at not only relaxing but also uplifting too that patients often have an almost instant relief from their stress.

There are three main ways which you can use oils to do a "spot repair" for stress. That is to relax you after a bad day for instance. The first is a warm bath with essential oils which will relax the muscles and slow down the heart rate and breathing but also calm the mind too.
The next is massage. This is wonderfully relaxing because the therapist will use very long slow movements which will still the mind. The massage also warms and kneads the muscles releasing toxins which are creating muscle stiffness and pain.

Evaporators in the room are lovely way to change the atmosphere and just bring a relaxing vibe to the room. The oils evaporate into the air and the chemical molecules travel up the nose and reach the limbic system of the brain, very quickly soothing the mind into a far more sedate state.

For long term stress I would suggest mixing oils into a cream or lotion which can be used as regularly as three times daily. By applying the smallest amount of cream to the inside of the arm the oils are able to absorb through the skin and into the blood stream. This means the oils are able to have an extremely targeted attack and maintain a good level of resistance over time.

Here are some ideas of oils to use:

Lavender and Camomile are extremely soothing and I would also want to add these into a blend. **Geranium** is extremely sedative but is uplifting too and really helps to build resilience to the feelings of worthlessness which stress can bring. **Bergamot** is like liquid sunshine and while calming it will also lift the spirits too.

If the body is under the rigors of stress for a long time there are some organs and glands which do not fare as well as others. The adrenal for instance can become completely depleted and I would suggest using **Mandarin** to support these. The liver too struggles to keep up with the pace and **Eucalyptus, Carrot and Peppermint really** help to invigorate this too.

Lastly I would consider using **Frankincense** to the blend so the breathing of the patient becomes slow and thus calming the heart rate too. Ultimately stress is the body's reaction to a situation that it does not want to be in. These essential oils will help a patient to relax but sooner or later they will need to address the problems facing them. In the meantime aromatherapy can really help the patient to deal with their stress.

How to treat diarrhea with aromatherapy?

While aromatherapy can offer some help to suffers or diarrhea, this is one condition which should be quickly taken to the doctors. It's a clear indication that something is going wrong with the body and so should not be ignored.

These are some oils which can help alleviate the symptoms:

Tea tree is by far the most effective method I know for killing bugs and germs. As a first line of defense I would pour a few drops of neat Tea tree oil into the inside of the wrist. This gives fast absorption into the blood stream and allows the essential oil to really start fighting any infection that might be the root of the problem.

Tea tree is antiviral, antiseptic and antibacterial and can address any underlying nasties which may be the root cause of the problem. The body very cleverly takes the effects of the oil which it needs and will eliminate anything which is surplus to requirement and reject it as waste. Given this then if root is not a nasty, the body simply will not use the Tea tree.

Ginger oil is a super oil for any condition where the body is struggling to cope with moisture.

Coriander and **Peppermint** are very good digestive oils and **Carrot seed** oil is calmative.

Camomile and **Rosemary** will both help with intestinal cramping (patients suffering from epilepsy should not use Rosemary as it can induce fits.)

It should also be borne in mind that diarrhea can often be a symptom of stress and while these oils will help stem the symptoms, it may be worth considering aromatherapy oils which can help to relax as well as treat the diarrhea.

These oils work particularly well used in a cream or lotion which can be applied to the inside of the wrist but also the abdomen to get a very fast absorption into the digestive tract.

Massaging the abdomen is very simple but it should be done with a very light touch. The purpose is really to lay the oils upon the skin to allow them to do their jobs. Massage is done in a clockwise direction in the shape of a square. Surrounding the belly button, do two strokes up, two strokes across the abdomen, two down the other side and then just one across the pelvis. Repeat until the oils have absorbed. This echoes the route of the food and as such any other problems lurking in the gut and allows the aromatherapy to cut right to the effects of the diarrhea.

How to treat earache with aromatherapy?

Treating earache with aromatherapy is simple and easy to do. It should however only be used as an emergency measure before getting to the doctors to have it checked out properly. It requires two lines of attack. The first is to treat any infection which may be causing earache. Since ear infections spread very quickly it is advisable to rub neat **Tea tree** around the front of the ear on the side of the face and then down the neck too.

Do not place oils inside the ear.

Secondly treat the pain and inflammation with **Lavender** and **Camomile**. **Camomile maroc** is very good here but if you use Camomile roman it has a stronger anti inflammatory qualities. It works well to mix these in a little bit of warmed vegetable oil and just rub around the outside of the ear. Work down the neck to stimulate the lymphatic nodes to start to fight any infection too.

For really painful episodes try soaking a flannel in warm water with these oils and then squeezing out. Lay the warm compress over the ear for about 20 minutes.

How to treat premenstrual syndrome with aromatherapy?

Aromatherapy is a wonderful way to treat premenstrual syndrome because it is pain relieving and relaxing.

Firstly I would suggest getting an oil which will balance out your hormones. **Rose** is wonderful as is **Geranium**, which is cheaper too.

Next consider the physical effects of the syndrome, bloating and swelling, pain and also in some cases heavy bleeding too.

The pain is best treated with as variety of oils, **Lavender** and **Camomile** will soothe tummy ache, for really searing pain I would consider **Camomile German** and also **Yarrow**.

The bloating which you feel comes from water retention. By using diuretic oils it allows the fluid to drain away but also reduces the pressure between the bladder and the uterus which is already full of blood. **Fennel, Juniper and Grapefruit** are all wonderful here and work remarkably quickly.

Emotionally some women can feel a little" delicate" (carefully put you notice!), again **Lavender, Camomile and Geranium** will all ease the emotional pressure I would also add **Bergamot and Clary sage** too.

Rose and Jasmine are wonderful tonics for the uterus; they will reduce clotting which can be a very bad source of pain.

PMS can be very often linked to some sort of pelvic infection which **Tea tree, Manuka** and **Kanuka** are all equipped to attack. For ongoing problems though it is advised that qualified medical attention is sought.

Lastly diet can really help alleviate menstrual symptoms. It is advised that both sugar and red meat are reduced during the week before menstruation.

While of course it is possible to use any of these oils in isolation to treat presenting symptoms a blend will work better. Massaging a small amount of the oils across the abdomen and small of the back will give the most amount of relief from pain. Dilute a blend of 3% essential oils to 97% carrier. **Evening primrose and Jasmine oils** both make marvelous additions to your premenstrual syndrome treatments here.

How to treat colds with aromatherapy?

As winter draws in it is worth checking out some aromatherapy treatments to keep colds and flu from your door. Here are my top ten oils for treating colds.

Tea tree – Is by far the most effective line of defense against any bugs which are brewing. Rub it on neat onto the skin or in the bath for 20 minutes. The oils penetrate through the skin and trigger the white cells of the immune system to combat the infection. It is also worth wiping down surfaces, door handles, light switches, etc when a bug is running through the house.

Lemon – This is a wonderful feeling in the sinuses when you have a blocked up nose. It cuts through catarrh and eases the pressure of cold headaches too. On top of this of course it is chock full of vitamin C.

Myrrh –The most wonderful decongestant. It is able to break the stickiest catarrh and move it right out of the sinus cavities and off the chest.

Ginger - This oil is a wonder for any conditions where the body struggles to control moisture. It balances the mucous membranes and eases the flow! Ginger also helps to regulate temperature so if the mercury is flying up the thermometer this oil will really help.

Eucalyptus - Even though this oil has very little power when it comes to fighting infection it is like a sledgehammer in clearing your nose. I find this most effective either in the bath or used as an inhalation to really make your nose run so you can get to sleep.

Myrtle - This is very gentle oil and is of particular help when treating children. It works on two levels, it will really help to calm a cough but also helps with how terribly upset they become too. This is a lovely oil to have.

Manuka – Many of you will recognize the name of the very expensive honey which has been harvested from bees who had fed on the manuka flowers. This is a very powerful antibacterial and again is great for battling bugs.

Kanuka – Often you will see this oil listed alongside Manuka. Recently though it was reclassified as belonging to an entirely different genus of plant. This is a serious warrior against infection and I tend to use it as my "go to" oil.

Ravensara – In among the list of very clinical scented oils is Ravensara, a lovely sharp fresh fragrance. This oil has even been found effective against strains of cholera and typhoid in trials.

Cedarwood atlas – In clinical trials this has proved to be the most effective oil in the treatment of infection. It is however very strong and should always be diluted.

How to treat flu with aromatherapy?

In the colder days of winter, aromatherapy offers a great deal of defence against colds and flu. As we turn on our heating to fight against the cold it provides the perfect breeding ground for bugs. Here are my top tips for staying healthy in the winter.

Tea tree is by far the most effective line of defence against any bugs which are brewing. Other great ones to try are **Manuka, Kanuka, Ravensara, Elemi and Niaouli.** Rub Tea tree neat onto the skin but all others will need to be diluted into some sort of carrier. You can use creams and lotions or any kind of vegetable oil will do. Use in a concentration of around 3% essential oils to 97% carrier (this need not be an exact science!)

For a really great way to get the oils into the system put some drops in your bath water and languish there for around 20 minutes. The oils penetrate through the skin and trigger white cells of the immune system to combat infection. It is also worth wiping down surfaces, door handles, light switches etc when a bug is running through the house.

For the misery of a blocked up nose it is worth making up a blend to rub on your face. **Lemon, Myrrh and Frankincense** all make wonderful decongestants and cut through catarrh.

Ginger; this oil is a wonderful choice for any conditions where the body is struggling to control moisture. In the case of flu of course is a runny nose and it balances the mucous membranes and eases the flow! It also works with the body to manage the hot and cold sweats which the body uses to purge itself of the infection. Ginger also helps to regulate temperature so if the mercury is flying up the thermometer this oil will really help.

Cedarwood atlas- In clinical trials Cedarwood proved to be the most effective oil in the treatment of infection. It fared very well against 3 different strains of stapphylococus, against influenza and also E coli. It is however very strong and should always be used diluted.

Coughs can be well managed using essential oils. For children I would suggest the use of **Myrtl. Inula** is a wonderful oil for the lungs and I have used it to great effect when I had pleurisy. Often with a cough there can be a difficulty to catch your breath, **Frankincense** is very good at decongesting the catarrh on the chest.

How to treat wounds with aromatherapy?

Aromatherapy is very effective in healing skin and wounds. It is important not to use oils on the broken area itself, rather allow the oils to work their magic from within. The oils absorb through the skin and into the blood stream and work with the body's natural processes to encourage healing.

Lavender oil is very good for treating pain of the initial injury. It is also the very best treatment for burns. Tests have shown that the healing capacity of the skin tissues is quickened radically with the use of this oil.

If there is a problem with excessive bleeding a compress using Geranium oil can help to stem the flow. This is best done using just a few drops of the oil into cold water and then making a compress on the wound. Not only will this clean the area but the combination of the drop in temperature and the oils make the capillaries shrink allowing less blood to flow.

Tea tree is effective in cleaning a wound and ensuring that no infection can get in.

Myrrh oil and **Galbanum** are extremely powerful skin healers and also have antiseptic qualities. These are very effective in cases where the skin has become weakened and frail.

When the wound has begun to heal **Jasmine** is wonderful oil for treating scarring. This is best applied daily for a period of around 4-6 weeks to really mend the skin and reducing marking.

How to treat muscle pain with aromatherapy?

Aromatherapy is best known for being used in massage and muscles absolutely adore the fuss! The muscles themselves are made up of complex bundles of fibers which send messages to and from the brain. The job of the muscles is not only to make our body move but also they are responsible for the heat we use in our body. They take nutrients from the blood and as they work they create waste product which is called lactic acid. The lymphatic system is responsible for moving this and sending it out of our bodies as waste. Sometimes though our bodies cannot keep up and so toxicity builds up inside the fibers. They are no longer able to slip easily over each other and they become painful to move.

Here are some oils which are effective in dealing with these problems:

Lavender is extremely useful for easing the pain as is **Geranium**. **Juniper** can alleviate the toxicity by breaking down the uric acid and flushing it out the system.

Black pepper and **marjoram** are superb oils for increasing circulation to the area, flushing it with oxygen which will also in turn help with the pain.

These combinations of oil will also work with pain which comes from conditions such as arthritis, rheumatism or fibromyalgia.

For nerve pain I would use **Rosemary oil** and for tendons I would use **Frankincense** to increase their elasticity and motility again.

There are also carrier oils which are far less dilute and make a lovely safe vehicle in which to transport your oils. **Borage and St John's Wort** are very effective. Use a dilution of 3% essential oils to 97% carrier. It is necessary to check with a doctor whether St John's Wort is safe if you are on any medication as it can neutralize some types of drugs.

Oils used in the bath are very effective but by far the best way of treating muscle pain with aromatherapy is with massage.

What is a good essential oil to treat Indigestion?

The best oil for treating indigestion is **Peppermint**. Just like your old gran always put mint sauce with her lamb it still is the best treatment to have. The reason that it works so well is it is able to break down fat to make it easier for the digestive system to process. Its lesser known sister S**pearmint** works effectively too.

Camomile is extremely good at easing the tightness of the pain if you have no Peppermint at hand.

Other digestive oils which can help are **Dill**, which also works very well for the effects of colic. Most usually this works best on babies and horses!

Many of the other spices which you find in curries too make excellent digestive aids. It do not only enhances the flavor of the food but also to soften the effects on the gut too. **Coriander, Cumin and Turmeric** are all digestive oils.

Peppermint does need to be diluted (as do all the oils listed here). Drop one drip of oil into a teaspoon of carrier (any vegetable oil out of the kitchen will do) and massage it onto the ribs over the pain. The oils absorb through the skin and into the blood stream and loosen the spasms causing the indigestion agony

How to treat menopause with aromatherapy?

The symptoms of menopause can be very unsettling but aromatherapy can offer a great helping hand. Clearing the underlying factors of this cannot be changed. The body alters as we get older and no longer need to reproduce. The hormonal changes and the effects which play in our day to day lives can be managed well using essential oils.

As the body ceases to manufacture oestrogen and progesterone so readily our skin begins to dry and our bones become more brittle. **Rose** oil is rich with oestrogol which makes a superb replacement for the system. This oil helps to regulate the waning periods and brings a flush back to the cheeks.

Hot flushes and night sweats are the demon menopausal visitors. **Clary sage** helps reduce the sweating and **Peppermint** eases the heat.

Mood swings can be a difficult part of the aging process and **Geranium** and **Ylang ylang** help steady the nerves and reduces stress.

The memory too can become a little stretched. **Rosewood and Rosemary** both help to focus the brain at a time where we are awash with hormones.

Libido can also change a great deal at this time. Some women feel liberated by the end of worry of pregnancy. Others feel far less sexy than they did. **Jasmine and sandalwood** blended with **Ylang ylang** really helps a women feel good again. Those whose libido has gone off the scale may find themselves suddenly out of step with their partner. **Marjoram** is an aphrodisiac- it quells libido and drive.

Each of these can be blended together into a cream or lotion to be used on a daily basis. This allows the body very slowly and gently to assimilate the changes. Alternatively they could be blended into a massage oil. **Evening Primrose** makes a beautiful choice here. Mix 3% essential oil to 97% carrier.

The oils can of course be added to the bath water for wonderfully luxurious soak (Rose and Jasmine are a bit expensive for that so use Geranium instead)

Lastly the most effective way to treat menopause with aromatherapy I find is to make the women look good. **Frankincense** blended into a moisturizer returns a richness and elasticity to her skin she may of said goodbye to years ago.

How to treat bruises with aromatherapy?

While aromatherapy can help heal bruises the plant choices recommended cross over into the world of herbals too.

Geranium oil works wonderfully to reduce the blood pressure around the injury and so reducing bruising. **Lavender** eases pain. Sometimes there can be swelling around the injury and we call this edema. Fennel oil makes a wonderful diuretic to flush out this extra fluid. The best way to treat a bruise is with regular cold water compresses. Drop a few drips of oil into cold water and then soak a towel in it. Place the compress over the affected area and the oils will absorb into the blood stream helping the bruise to dissipate.

It is also worth getting some arnica gel and some witch hazel. These are easily obtained from the chemist and also plant extracts. Blend geranium oil into the gel or the witch hazel for an extremely potent treatment for your bruising.

How to treat burns with aromatherapy?

The basis of aromatherapy was built on the result of an accident with a burn. The observations of which were gained from it lead us to the complex art of aromatherapy as we know it today. By far the most effective treatment for burns is to apply neat **lavender oil** onto the affected part.

In the late 1920s a scientist by the name of Dr Jean Valnet was conducting experiments in his lab. Distracted he caught his hand on a Bunsen burner and suffered a terrible burn. In agony he plunged his hand into the first vat of liquid he could find. Luckily for him contained within was lavender oil. Never since have we found a more efficient mode of healing for burns. Neither would we need to. It is so efficient.

Always treat burns by first running them under the cold tap for a few minutes to take the heat out of the burn. Next, sprinkle liberally with neat lavender oil.

I have also found aloe Vera gel to be very soothing to burns too. The two aromatherapy products work well together.

How to treat nausea with aromatherapy?

There are four main oils in aromatherapy to treat nausea. These are camomile, mandarin, peppermint and ginger.

I would advocate Mandarin for used for morning sickness. Replace camomile and peppermint oils with camomile and peppermint tea and ginger oil with ginger biscuits.

These oils work very well for nausea from motion sickness too.

For stomach bugs I would consider also adding tea tree oil to kill and infection which may be causing the symptoms.

Aromatherapy works with essential oils absorbing through the skin and into the blood stream. The best application of these would be to add a few drops to a table spoon of carrier oil and then massage gently over the abdomen.

How to end an aromatherapy session?

The end of an aromatherapy session can almost feel like a wrench to patients as they force themselves to open their eyes to the world. A gentle transition from asleep to awake is necessary.

Ensure they are well covered with a towel to keep them warm. Many patients will have drifted into semi sleep so gently tell them you will leave them there until they are ready to get up.

Wait for them to stir and then be ready with a cleansing and grounding glass of water.

If you have been administering aromatherapy to yourself ensure your hands are well washed and you drink lots of water.

Remember too, that the oils will take a good twenty minutes to absorb through the skin to ensure enough time has elapsed before you bath or shower.

.

www.ingramcontent.com/pod-product-compliance
Lightning Source LLC
Chambersburg PA
CBHW070304290526
45791CB00003B/1078